Published By Adam Gilbin

@ Harris Hile

The Pegan Diet: The Complete and Easy Cookbook

for Beginners Plus 150+ Delicious Recipes

All Right RESERVED

ISBN 978-1-990666-77-3

I0558145

TABLE OF CONTENTS

Strawberry Coconut Smoothie

Ingredients:

- 1 frozen banana, sliced

- 1 cup coconut milk

- 1 tsp vanilla extract

- 2 cups frozen strawberries

- 1 scoop collagen peptides (discretionary, search for veggie lover choices if necessary)

Directions:

1. Add every one of the fixings to a blender and mix at a high velocity until totally smooth.

Fall Smoothie

Ingredients:

- 1 frozen banana, sliced

- 2 tsp pumpkin pie zest or 1 tsp cinnamon and 1 tsp of ginger

- ¼ cup pumpkin puree

- 1 cup coconut milk

- 1 cup ice

Directions:

1. Add every one of the fixings to a blender that can hack ice and mix until the substance have a smooth consistency.
2. Serve immediately.

Dark Chocolate–Raspberry Shortbread Bars

Ingredients:

For shortbread:

- ½ teaspoon vanilla extract

- 2 cups (193 g) blanched almond flour

- Pinch sea salt

- 6 tablespoons (¾ stick; 84 g) pastured butter, at room temperature

- ¼ cup (80 g) honey

For chocolate-date layer:

- 3 tablespoons (42 g) pastured butter, at room temperature

- Pinch sea salt

- 20 ounces (560 g) pitted Medjool dates

- ¼ cup (22 g) cacao powder

For topping:

- 1 cup (125 g) fresh raspberries

- 1¾ ounces (50 g) 85% or 100% dark chocolate, melted

Directions:

1. To make the shortbread: Preheat the oven to 350°F (180°C, or gas mark 4). Line an 8 × 8-inch (20 × 20 cm) baking pan with parchment paper.

2. In the bowl of a stand mixer fitted with the paddle attachment, or in a large bowl and using a hand mixer, beat the butter, honey, and vanilla on medium speed until light and fluffy.

3. Add the almond flour and salt (up to ¼ teaspoon if the butter is unsalted) and mix until there is no dry flour left.

4. Press the shortbread dough into the prepared pan. Use a pastry roller, or your hands, to flatten the dough into a smooth and even layer.
5. Use a fork or a chopstick to poke holes across the shortbread to ensure the dough cooks in the center as well as around the edges.
6. Bake the shortbread for 22 to 24 minutes until the top is a light golden brown.
7. Remove from the oven and let cool fully before topping with the chocolate-date layer.
8. To make the chocolate-date layer: Place the dates in a medium-size bowl and cover them with boiling water.
9. Let soak for about 5 minutes. Drain all the water from the dates and transfer to a food processor.
10. Add the cacao powder, butter, and salt. Process for 3 to 4 minutes, stopping to scrape

the mixture from the sides about every minute or so.

11. The mixture is ready when there are no pieces of date visible and the mixture is smooth and caramel-like. If necessary, add 1 to 2 tablespoons (15 to 30 ml) of hot water to reach the desired texture.

12. Once the shortbread has fully cooled, spread the chocolate-date mixture over the top and use wet hands to flatten it into a smooth layer.

13. To make the topping: Top the date layer with the raspberries and drizzle with the melted dark chocolate.

14. Chill thoroughly before cutting and serving.

15. Refrigerate leftovers tightly wrapped, or in an airtight container, for up to 4 days.

Maple-Pegan Macaroons

Ingredients:

- ½ teaspoon vanilla extract

- 2 cups (170 g) finely shredded unsweetened coconut

- ½ cup (55 g) finely chopped pecans, plus more for garnish (optional)

- 3 ounces (85 g) unsweetened chocolate

- ⅓ cup (107 g) maple syrup

- 1 teaspoon grass-fed gelatin

- ½ teaspoon almond exact

Directions:

1. Preheat the oven to 350°F (180°C, or gas mark 4). Line a baking sheet with parchment paper or a silicone baking mat.

2. In a medium-size bowl, whisk the egg whites and maple syrup until very foamy. It isn't necessary to whisk to form peaks, like in a meringue, but the mixture should be lightened.

3. Add the gelatin, almond extract, and vanilla and whisk well.

4. Add the coconut and pecans and stir to evenly coat with the egg white mixture.

5. Use a rounded tablespoon or cookie scoop to scoop and compact the coconut batter, pressing it to hold it together well, before placing it on the prepared baking sheet. Repeat to make 20 cookies.

6. Bake the cookies for 16 to 18 minutes until lightly browned on top. Let cool fully.

7. In a double boiler, melt the unsweetened chocolate.

8. Dip the base of each cookie into the melted chocolate to coat, placing them on a piece of wax paper to set.

9. Use a fork to drizzle any remaining

10. Chocolate on the tops of the cookies. Sprinkle the cookies with additional chopped pecans (if using).

Saffron Carrots With Apricots And Orange

Ingredients:

- 25 g dried apricots

- 1 tbsp. olive oil

- 1 pinch saffron thread

- 1 stem parsley

- 400 g carrots (4 carrots)

- 100 ml classic vegetable broth

- 1 shallot

- 1 orange

Salt pepper

Directions:

1. Wash the carrots before cut them into 5 mm thick slices.

2. Peel and cleave finely the shallot and dice the apricots.

3. In a pot, heat the oil and sauté the shallot for 2-3 minutes over medium hotness.

4. Cook for 1 moment in the wake of adding the carrots.

5. Season with salt and pepper and odd the apricots and saffron.

6. Squeeze the orange. Pour the stock and squeezed orange over the carrots and cook for 8-9 minutes, covered, until they mineral delicate to the bite.

7. Meanwhile, wash the parsley, shake it out, eliminate the leaves, cleave it up, and blend it into the carrots.

8. Serve hot or cold, preparing with salt and pepper.

Fruit And Nut Salad

Ingredients:

- 1 tablespoon chopped fresh mint leaves

- 1 / 4 teaspoon salt

- 2 cups sliced strawberries

- 2 cups blueberries

- 2 cups cubed watermelon

- 1 / 2 cup chopped toasted hazelnuts

- 1 tablespoon hazelnut oil

- 2 tablespoons olive oil

- 2 tablespoons lemon juice

- 2 tablespoons chopped fresh basil leaves

- 1 / 4 cup toasted pine nuts

Directions:

1. In a large bowl, combine hazelnut oil, olive oil, lemon juice, basil, mint, and salt and whisk until combined.

2. Add fruits and toss gently until coated. Top with nuts and serve immediately.

Basic Vegetable Stock

Ingredients:

- 1 pound celery, roughly chopped

- 1 1 / 2 gallons water

- 1 cup chopped parsley stems

- 4 sprigs fresh thyme

- 2 bay leaves

- 2 pounds yellow onions, peeled and roughly chopped

- 1 pound carrots, peeled and roughly chopped

- 15 peppercorns

Directions:

1. Place onions, carrots, celery, and water in a large stockpot over medium heat; bring to a

simmer and cook, uncovered, for $1 \frac{1}{2}$ hours.

2. Add parsley stems, thyme, bay leaves, and peppercorns, and continue to simmer, uncovered, for 45 minutes.

3. Remove from heat and strain stock. Discard solids.

4. Stock can be refrigerated for two to four days or frozen for up to three months.

Italian Dressing

Ingredients:

- 1 teaspoon dried oregano

- 1 / 2 teaspoon salt

- 1 / 2 teaspoon ground black pepper

- 1 / 2 cup extra-virgin olive oil

- 1 / 3 cup apple cider vinegar

- 1 / 2 teaspoon dry mustard

- 1 teaspoon lemon juice

- 2 cloves garlic, peeled and chopped

Directions:

1. Place all INGREDIENTS: except olive oil in a blender.

2. With the blender running on a medium setting, slowly pour in oil. Blend until smooth.
3. Serve immediately on salad or cover and store in the refrigerator for up to seven days.

French Dressing

Ingredients:

- 2 tablespoons Homemade Ketchup (see recipe in Chapter 9)

- 1 tablespoon Dijon mustard

- 2 1 / 2 tablespoons maple syrup

- 1 / 2 cup olive oil

- 1 / 2 teaspoon smoked paprika

- 1 / 4 teaspoon salt

- 1 / 8 teaspoon ground white pepper

- 1 small onion, peeled and finely chopped

- 2 cloves garlic, peeled and minced

- 1 / 4 cup apple cider vinegar

- 1 tablespoon lemon juice

- 2 tablespoons tomato paste

Directions:

1. Combine all INGREDIENTS: in a food processor or blender. Cover and blend until smooth.

2. Cover and refrigerate for 2–3 hours to let flavors blend.

3. Store tightly covered in the refrigerator for up to five days.

Honey-Lemon Dressing

Ingredients:

- 1 tablespoon honey

- ½ teaspoon chopped thyme

- ¼ cup extra-virgin olive oil

- 2tablespoon plus two teaspoons fresh lemon juice

- 1 teaspoon finely grated lemon zest

- Kosher salt and freshly ground pepper

Directions:

1. In a little bowl, mix the lemon juice, lemon zest, honey, and thyme until well combined.
2. Add the olive oil and season with salt and pepper after whisking it in.

Avocado & Black Bean Egg Wrapped Breakfast Burrito

Ingredients:

- ¼ cup shredded cheddar cheese(25 g)

- ¼ cup black beans(40 g)

- ¼ cup onion(40 g), cooked

- ¼ cup bell pepper(25 g), cooked

- 2slices avocado

- 2 eggs

- Salt, to taste

- 2tablespoon shredded parmesan cheese

- ½ tablespoon butter

Directions:

1. Whisk together the eggs, salt, and Parmesan in a medium mixing bowl until thoroughly blended.

2. Pouring the egg mixture into a medium saucepan with the butter already melted over medium heat.

3. Allow the egg to cook until it begins to solidify, then fill the middle of the egg wrap with cheddar cheese, black beans, onions, and peppers.

4. Cooking for another 3 minutes, or up to the egg is thoroughly cooked and the cheese is melted, covered with a lid.

5. Remove the avocados from the pan and add them.

6. To make a burrito, fold in the left and right edges of the egg wrap, then roll from the bottom to the top.

7. Enjoy!

Spiced Up Lettuce Chicken

Ingredients:

- Pinch of sugar

- Lettuce as needed

- Fresh coriander leaves

- Jalapeno chillies, sliced

- Fresh tomato slices for garnish

- 1 pound chicken breast, cut into strips

- Splash of olive oil

- 1 red onion, finely sliced

- 14 ounces tomatoes

- 1 teaspoon chipotle, chopped

- ½ teaspoon cumin

- Lime wedges

Directions:

1. Take a non-stick frying pan and place it over medium heat
2. Add oil and heat it up
3. Add chicken and cook until brown
4. Keep the chicken on the side
5. Add tomatoes, sugar, chipotle, cumin to the same pan and simmer for 25 minutes until you have a nice sauce
6. Add chicken into the sauce and cook for 5 minutes
7. Transfer the mix to another place
8. Use lettuce wraps to take a portion of the mixture and serve with a squeeze of lemon
9. Enjoy!

Parsley Chicken Breast

Ingredients:

- ½ teaspoon salt

- ½ teaspoon red pepper flakes, crushed

- 2 tomatoes, sliced

- 1 tablespoon dry parsley

- 1 tablespoon dry basil

- 4 chicken breast halves, boneless and skinless

Directions:

1. Preheat your oven to 350 degrees F
2. Take a 9x13 inch baking dish and grease it up with cooking spray
3. Sprinkle 1 tablespoon of parsley, 1 teaspoon of basil, and spread the mixture over your baking dish

4. Arrange the chicken breast halves over the dish and sprinkle garlic slices on top
5. Take a small bowl and add 1 teaspoon parsley, 1 teaspoon of basil, salt, basil, red pepper, and mix well. Pour the mixture over the chicken breast
6. Top with tomato slices and cover, bake for 25 minutes
7. Remove the cover and bake for 15 minutes more
8. Serve and enjoy!

Broccoli Salad With Creamy Ginger Mustard Dressing

Ingredients:

- 1–2 bulbs scallions, chopped

- 8 oz shirataki noodles

- Creamy ginger salad dressing

- 4 slices crispy bacon (optional)

- 6–8 oz sugar snap or snow peas, remove the tips and tough string that run through them

- 1–2 whole ripe avocados, sliced

- 3–4 whole soft warm boiled eggs, divided in half

- 1 lb broccolini (discard bottom third of stems then split in half) or broccoli (cut into florets)

Directions:

1. Start boiling a large pot of water.

2. Make the ginger salad dressing unless you have some dressing stored in your fridge.

3. Cook the bacon until it is crispy then prepare the noodles, scallions, and avocados.

4. Once the water is boiling, lower the heat down to medium low and add the eggs to the water. Cook the eggs uncovered for 6 ½ minutes, gently moving the eggs now and again to ensure that the eggs cook fully but remain soft.

5. Once the eggs are cooked, submerge them in cold water until cool.

6. While the eggs are cooling, blanch the vegetables. If using broccolini, blanch in hot water for 2 minutes; if using broccoli, then blanch for 60–90 seconds. The snap peas can be blanched for 30 seconds to a minute.

7. Once all the vegetables are blanched, add them to cold water to stop the cooking process, then drain them thoroughly. All vegetables should remain crispy but also tender.

8. In a large serving bowl, add all the vegetables, the halved soft eggs, and crispy bacon the drizzle with the creamy ginger salad dressing.

9. Salad is best served at room temperature or chilled.

Kale Salad With Almonds And Lime

Ingredients:

- 1 tbsp coconut oil

- ½-inch piece of ginger, chopped

- ½ lime, juiced

- 1 clove garlic, pressed

- ½ cup almonds, soaked at least 8 hours

- 3–4 kale leaves, remove the stems

- 2 tbsp olive oil

Directions:

1. Chop the kale into bite-sized pieces.
2. Add two cups of water to a pot to boil.
3. Drain the almonds then add them to the boiling water for 30 seconds. Remove and add to cold water immediately to make it easier to

remove the skins simply by pinching them off one by one.

4. Once the skin has been removed, chop the almonds finely.

5. Add some coconut oil to a pan over medium heat then add the garlic and ginger before cooking for 2 minutes.

6. Add the kale leaves to the mixture and cook until softened. Add a tablespoon of water to prevent the leaves from burning.

7. Once the kale is soft, remove it from the heat.

8. Add the lime juice and olive oil to a small bowl and whisk until fully emulsified.

9. Mix the kale mixture, dressing, and almonds then toss before serving.

Crumbled Tempe Sausage

Ingredients:

- 1 level teaspoon of Worcestershire sauce

- 1 teaspoon of onion powder

- 1half of a teaspoon of oregano

- 1 teaspoon of garlic powder

- a half teaspoon of sage and a quarter teaspoon of black pepper

- ¼ teaspoon of thyme

- 1 and one-half cups of water

- 1 box of tempeh, plain and unflavored, weighing 8 ounces;

- 2 tablespoons of soy sauce

- 1 level teaspoon of paprika

- 1 tablespoon of oil

- A pinch or two of chili flakes

Directions:

1. Crumble the tempeh in the pan that it will be cooked in.

2. Give everything, with the exception of the oil, a good stir after adding the water and the extra INGREDIENTS:.

3. Bring to a simmer over a heat that is medium-low in intensity. Continue to boil the tempeh until it has completely absorbed all of the liquid.

4. After adding the oil, give the mixture a toss and continue to cook it for approximately five more minutes over medium heat. (If you have cut oil out of your diet, you may omit this step; the sausage will still have a fantastic flavor even if you do so.)

Baked Sausage Patties

Ingredients:

- 2 tablespoons of soy sauce

- 1 tablespoon of maple syrup

- 2 teaspoons of garlic powder

- 1 teaspoon of sage

- 2 teaspoons of onion powder

- 1 tablespoon of sage

- 2 tablespoons of liquid, which was retained from the can

- 1 can of pinto beans, from which the liquid was drained

- 3 tablespoons of breadcrumbs

- 1 tsp. Of smoked paprika

- One-fourth of a teaspoon of thyme

- One-half of a teaspoon of rosemary

- Freshly ground black pepper to taste

- A teaspoon of dried chili flakes

Directions:

1. Preheat the oven to 475 degrees. Set the broiler to high.
2. Cover a baking sheet with parchment paper before using it.
3. The pinto beans and the liquid that was saved from the can are combined in a blender.
4. Don't turn into complete mush; there should still be some substance.
5. In a mixing bowl, combine the pinto beans and the other INGREDIENTS:.

6. Shape into patties. Put the baking sheet that is covered in parchment paper into the oven.
7. It is recommended that the patties be baked for around 16 minutes total, with one flip occurring every 7-8 minutes. Enjoy!

Citrus Pear And Cabbage Smoothie

Ingredients:

- 30 g organic currants

- 2-3 organic pears

- 1 banana

- 500 ml organic almond milk with no added sugar

- 1 teaspoon grated ginger

- 1 organic orange

- 30 g organic raspberries

- 30 g organic blackberries

- orange peel

- 100 g leaves black cabbage

- 2 tablespoons chia seeds

- ice cubes

Directions:

1. Wash the cabbage leaves well and cut them into pieces, wash all the fruit and peel the pears removing the inner seeds.

2. Peel and cut the banana and orange into pieces then put all the INGREDIENTS: in the blender and operate until smooth.

3. Add the orange zest, blend and enjoy!

Tropical Smoothie

Ingredients:

- 6 fresh mint leaves

- 2 tablespoons agave syrup

- ice cubes

- 240 ml of coconut water

- 2 organic cucumbers

- 150 g frozen pineapple in pieces

- juice of 1 lime

Directions:

1. Peel the cucumbers then cut them into pieces (if you prefer you can leave the peel on as well because it contains many minerals and vitamins), wash the mint leaves and put the

INGREDIENTS: in the blender glass, add half of the water and operate.

2. Gradually add all the coconut water and then serve over ice!

Mint And Chocolate Cheesecake Bites

Ingredients:

For chocolate cups:

- ⅓ cup coconut oil, melted

- ½ cup and 2 tbsp cocoa powder

- ¼ cup maple syrup

- Pinch of salt

For mint cheesecake filling:

- 2 cups cashews, absorbed water for two hours first, then, at that point, drained

- ½ cup pressed mint leaves (around 15 to 20 twigs of favored mint) 3 tbsp lemon juice

- ½ cup coconut oil, melted

- ½ cup maple syrup

- Touch of salt

- ½ tsp spirulina (discretionary, for color)

Directions:

For cups:

1. Add the coconut oil, salt, maple syrup, and cocoa powder to a bowl and rush until the consistency appears as though softened chocolate.

2. Apply 2 tablespoons of the combination to the sides of the cupcake case until it is totally coated.

3. Once covered, hold the case topsy turvy over a bowl until the overabundance combination has trickled from it.

4. Once all the cupcake cases are covered add them to a plate straight up and freeze for around 30 minutes.

For filling:

1. While the chocolate cases are freezing start on the filling.

2. Add all the filling fixings to a blender and mix until totally smooth.

3. Add the smooth combination to a channeling pack (or a plastic sack with a corner cut away.)

4. Remove the frozen cups from the cooler and line in the topping off to their edge.

5. Freeze the entire treat for an additional 30 minutes to make it more straightforward to eliminate the cupcake cases.

6. Keep frozen until around 10-15 minutes prior to serving.

7. They can keep going for around fourteen days in the freezer.

8. Serve with some whipped coconut cream, sprinkled with nuts, and have a few new berries on the side.

Chocolate And Coconut Macaroons

Ingredients:

- 3 eggs, beaten

- 3 cup coconut chips, unsweetened

- 6 tbsp coconut oil

- ¼ cup and 2 tbsp warm water

- Stevia to taste

- ⅓ cup crude cacao powder (optional)

- Any seasoned concentrate (optional)

Directions:

1. Preheat the stove to 400 °F.
2. Add the warm water, dissolved oil, and coconut pieces to a bowl and mix until the drops are totally saturated.

In a new bowl, blend the eggs and stevia well. Add the egg combination to the coconut drop combination and blend well.

3. Split the combination fifty-fifty and add cocoa to one half.

4. Possibly do this in the event that you need a chocolate flavor.

5. Make sure to add a couple of additional drops of stevia to this blend, as it will be more bitter.

6. Scoop a little piece of the combination and add it to an ungreased treat sheet. You can smooth it with your fingers or with a fork or leave it round.

7. Bake for 12-15 minutes. Allow them to cool before eating.

8. These likewise freeze all around well yet delay until they are cooled prior to adding them to the freezer.

Superfoods Dark Chocolate Bark

Ingredients:

- 2 tablespoons (14 g) chopped pecans

- 2 tablespoons (16 g) pumpkin seeds

- 1 tablespoon (10 g) hemp seeds

- 6 ounces (170 g) 85% or higher dark chocolate

- 1 tablespoon (14 g) coconut oil

- ½ cup (90 g) pomegranate arils, divided

Directions:

1. Line a small baking sheet with parchment paper. Set aside.

2. In a double boiler, melt the chocolate and coconut oil, stirring until the mixture is smooth and fully melted. Stir in ¼ cup (45 g) of the pomegranate arils. Pour the chocolate

mixture onto the prepared baking sheet and spread into a large rectangle.

3. Sprinkle the top of the chocolate with the remaining ¼ cup (45 g) of pomegranate arils, as well as the pecans and seeds.

4. Refrigerate for about 20 minutes to set the chocolate, then break it into smaller pieces.

5. Keep refrigerated in an airtight container for about 1 week, or freeze for up to 3 months. Enjoy right out of the freezer to keep from melting.

No-Bake Cookie Dough Bars

Ingredients:

For cookie dough:

- ½ teaspoon sea salt

- 1 vanilla bean, scraped (reserve the pod for another use, like in smoothies)

- 1½ ounces (42 g) 85% to 90% dark chocolate, chopped

- Coarse sea salt, for garnish (optional)

- ¾ cup (90 g) raw buckwheat groats

- 1 cup (260 g) cashew butter

- ¼ cup (80 g) maple syrup

- 2 tablespoons (28 g) coconut oil, melted

For cashew fudge:

- 2 tablespoons (33 g) cashew butter

- 1½ ounces (42 g) 85% to 90% dark chocolate, chopped

- Line a standard loaf pan with parchment paper. Set aside.

Directions:

1. To make the cookie dough: In a blender, process the buckwheat groats into a fine flour. Set aside.

2. In a medium-size bowl, combine the cashew butter, maple syrup, melted coconut oil, sea salt, and scraped vanilla bean seeds. Stir the INGREDIENTS: well to combine.

3. Add the buckwheat flour and dark chocolate. Stir to combine until no dry flour remains. Press the cookie dough into the prepared loaf pan in an even layer.

4. To make the cashew fudge: In a small saucepan over very low heat, or in a double boiler, combine the cashew butter and dark chocolate. Cook for about 5 minutes, stirring to mix the INGREDIENTS: until fully melted, being careful not to scorch the chocolate. Spread the fudge over the cookie dough in an even layer. Sprinkle with coarse sea salt (if using).

5. Freeze the cookie dough bars for 30 minutes to set. Remove the bars from the freezer and cut into slices. To cut the bars without the chocolate cracking, let them sit at room temperature for 10 minutes to soften the fudge layer before cutting into them.

Teriyari Tuna With Ginger And Vegetables

Ingredients:

- 2 cloves garlic

- 1 tbsp. coconut oil

- 1tbsp. fresh ginger

- 1 red pepper

- 1 yellow pepper

- 1 carrot

- 400 g tuna fillet, cut into 4 pieces 50

- ml reduced sodium soy sauce 50 ml of sake

- 200 g fresh snow peas

- 2 tbsps. mirin

- 1 tbsp. granulated sugar

Directions:

1. Clean, wash and dry all the vegetables.

2. Thinly cut the peppers and the snow peas and cut into strips the carrot.

3. Chop finely the garlic and the new ginger.

4. Bring the soy sauce, purpose, mirin and sugar ta bubble in a saucepan.

5. Cook over medium-high hotness for around 5 minutes until the sauce has thickened.

6. Eliminate from heat, put half of the sauce in a bowl and keep warm.

7. Heat a huge non-stick skillet over medium-high hotness and add the coconut oil, ginger, and garlic.

8. Cook momentarily, mixing, until fragrant, then, at that point, add the snow peas, peppers and carrots; cook 4 minutes, mixing, until the vegetables are more delicate and put them, covered, aside.

9. Meanwhile, barbecue the fish on a hotness source, flipping and brushing with half of the sauce, until brilliant brown and marginally pink in the middle (around 3 minutes for every side).

10. Divide the vegetable combination into 4 plates and present with a piece of fish for each and shower with the leftover sauce.

Roasted Vegetable Stock

Ingredients:

- 3 medium rutabagas, quartered

- 3 medium bell peppers, seeded and halved

- 2 medium shallots, peeled

- 1 medium head garlic

- 1 medium bunch fresh thyme

- 1 medium bunch parsley

- 3 medium carrots, peeled and coarsely chopped

- 3 medium parsnips, peeled and coarsely chopped

- 3 large onions, peeled and quartered

- 3 whole medium turnips

- 5 quarts water

Directions:

1. Preheat oven to 425°F. Line a 9" × 13" baking pan with parchment paper.

2. Arrange all the vegetables and herbs in the pan and roast for 30 minutes or until browned.

3. Flip vegetables halfway through.

4. Add vegetables to a 6-quart slow cooker. Add 5 quarts water and cover.

5. Cook on low for 8–10 hours. Strain stock, discarding the solids.

6. Freeze or refrigerate stock and use within one to two weeks.

Mushroom Stock

Ingredients:

- 1 large onion, peeled and sliced

- 1 large leek (white part only)

- 1 medium stalk celery, sliced

- 2 ounces dried shiitake mushrooms

- 1 tablespoon minced garlic

- 1 1 / 2 teaspoons black peppercorns

- 3 / 4 teaspoon dried sage

- 1 quart water

- 12 ounces white mushrooms

- 6 parsley stems (with leaves)

- 3 / 4 teaspoon dried thyme leaves

- 1 / 2 teaspoon ground black pepper

Directions:

1. Combine all INGREDIENTS: except ground pepper in a 6-quart slow cooker; cover and cook on low for 6–8 hours.

2. Strain, discarding solids; season with ground pepper.

3. Serve immediately, refrigerate and use within one to two weeks, or freeze up to several months.

Cauliflower "Rice" Salad

Ingredients:

- 2 medium carrots, peeled and shredded

- 1 / 3 cup finely chopped dill pickle

- 1 / 3 cup extra-virgin olive oil

- 1 tablespoon maple syrup

- 1 tablespoon chopped fresh dill

- 1 / 4 teaspoon salt

- 1 / 8 teaspoon ground black pepper

- 1 medium head cauliflower, shredded

- 4 tablespoons lemon juice, divided

- 1 tablespoon coconut oil

- 4 medium stalks celery, sliced

- 1 medium yellow bell pepper, seeded and chopped

Directions:

1. Toss shredded cauliflower with 1 tablespoon lemon juice.
2. Heat coconut oil in medium skillet over medium heat.
3. Add shredded cauliflower and cook for 1–2 minutes or until crisp-tender.
4. Scrape cauliflower into a large bowl and set aside to cool for 15 minutes.
5. Stir celery, bell pepper, carrots, and dill pickle into cauliflower.
6. In a small bowl, combine olive oil, remaining 3 tablespoons lemon juice, maple syrup, dill, salt, and black pepper and mix well. Pour over salad and stir to coat.
7. Cover and chill for 1–3 hours before serving.

Spicy Sweet Cucumber Salad

Ingredients:

- 1 tablespoon maple syrup

- 1 teaspoon sesame oil

- 1 / 4 teaspoon crushed red pepper flakes

- 1 / 2 medium onion, peeled and thinly sliced

- 2 medium cucumbers, peeled and thinly sliced

- 3 / 4 teaspoon salt

- 1 / 4 cup apple cider vinegar

Directions:

1. In a large shallow container or on a large baking sheet, spread cucumbers in a single layer and sprinkle with salt.
2. Allow to sit at least 10 minutes.

3. Drain excess water from cucumbers. Transfer cucumbers to a medium bowl.

4. In a small bowl, whisk together vinegar, maple syrup, oil, and red pepper flakes.

5. Pour dressing over cucumbers, add onion, and toss gently.

6. Allow to sit at least 10 minutes before serving to allow flavors to mingle.

Beef Stew With Carrots & Potatoes

Ingredients:

- 7 garlic cloves, peeled and crushed

- 2 tblsp balsamic vinaigrette

- 1½ tablespoons tomato paste

- ¼ cup all-purpose flour

- 2 cups dry red wine

- 2 cups beef broth

- 2 cups water

- 1 bay leaf

- ½ teaspoon dried thyme

- 1½ teaspoons sugar

- 3 pound boneless, well-marbled beef chuck, cut into 112-inch chunks

- salt (two tablespoons)

- 3teaspoon black pepper, freshly ground

- 2tablespoons extra virgin olive oil

- 3medium yellow onions, roughly chopped into 1-inch slices

- Cut four large carrots into 1-inch slices on a diagonal and place them in a bowl.

- 1 pound halved baby yukon white boiling potatoes

- For garnishes, use freshly cut parsley.

Directions:
1. A lower-middle rack in the oven should be preheated to 325 degrees Fahrenheit.

2. Pat the meat dry before seasoning it with salt and pepper. In a big Dutch oven or heavy soup pot, heat 1 tablespoon olive oil over medium-high heat until hot and shimmering.

3. The meat should be browned in three batches, with one tablespoon of additional oil in each, for about five minutes each. Avoid crowding the pan when searing the meat, and don't rotate it until a nice brown crust has formed.) Set the meat aside in a large plate.

4. Using a wooden spoon, scrape the brown bits from the bottom of the pan, then add the onions, garlic, and balsamic vinegar after about 5 minutes of cooking. After the tomato paste has been added, cook for an additional minute. Season the meat with the flour and return it to the pan with the juices.

5. Stirring with a wooden spoon for 1 -2 minutes until the flour is fully dissolved. In a large mixing bowl, combine the wine, beef broth,

water, bay leaf, thyme, and sugar. Scrape the pan with a woodening spoon as the mixture comes to a boil. Place the covered saucepan in the preheated oven for two hours.

6. After cooking in the oven, add the potatoes and carrots to the saucepan. Remove from oven and allow to cool before serving.

7. Remove the bay leaf, taste, and season to taste. Keep the stew at room temperature for a few hours before refrigerating it overnight or until serving. This stew's taste improves if cooked a day ahead. Reheat at 350°F or on medium heat with the lid on.

8. Garnish with fresh parsley if preferred.

Mongolian Beef

Ingredients:

- 2 teaspoons minced fresh ginger

- 2tablespoon minced garlic

- 1/3 cup low-sodium light soy sauce

- 1/3 cup liquid

- 1/2 cup sugar (dark brown)

- 4 scallions stalks, cut into 2-inch chunks, green portions only

- Flank steak, 1 pound

- A quarter cup of cornstarch

- A quarter cup of canola oil

Directions:

1. After slicing the flank steak against the grain, fry it in a Ziploc bag with cornstarch .After pushing the steak around in the bag to ensure that it is fully covered with cornstarch, leave it aside to settle.

2. Heat the canola oil in a broad frying pan over medium-high heat.Remove any excess corn starch from the steak before cooking it for 1 minute on each side in the pan.

3. Cook the steak in stages if your pan isn't big enough to fit it all in at once. You want a good sear on your steak, not steam, so don't push it in.

4. When the steak is done, remove it from the pan.

5. Remove the ginger and garlic from the fire after 10 to 15 seconds of sautéing.Serve with rice or noodles, and if preferred, sprinkle with sesame seeds or other toppings.To thicken

the sauce, reintroduce the meat and simmer for another 20-30 seconds.

6. If the sauce isn't thick enough, combine 1 tablespoon cornstarch with 1 tablespoon water and mix to dissolve the cornstarch before adding it to the pan.

7. Stir in the green onions and heat for a few more seconds to incorporate them into the dish.

8. Serve at once.

Tasty Grilled Lime Shrimp

Ingredients:

- 1 lime, juiced

- ½ cup olive oil

- 3 tablespoons Cajun seasoning

- 1 pound medium shrimp, peeled and deveined

Directions:

1. Take a re-sealable zip bag and add lime juice, Cajun seasoning, olive oil
2. Add shrimp and shake it well, let it marinate for 20 minutes
3. Preheat your outdoor grill to medium heat
4. Lightly grease the grate
5. Remove shrimp from marinade and cook for 2 minutes per side Serve and enjoy!

Tasty Coconut And Hazelnut Haddock

Ingredients:

- 1 cup coconut, shredded and unsweetened

- ¼ cup hazelnuts, ground

- Salt to taste

- Some cooked spinach

- 4 haddock fillets, 5 ounces each, boneless

- 2 tablespoons coconut oil, melted

Directions:

1. Preheat your oven to 400 degrees F
2. Line a baking sheet with parchment paper
3. Keep it on the side
4. Pat fish fillets with a paper towel and season with salt

70

5. Take a bowl and stir in hazelnuts and shredded coconut
6. Drag fish fillets through the coconut mix until both sides are coated well
7. Transfer to a baking dish
8. Brush with coconut oil
9. Bake for about 12 minutes until flaky
10. Serve over a bed of cooked spinach and enjoy!

Sugar-Free Berry Jam

Ingredients:

- 2 tsp chia seeds, ground

- ½–1 tsp lemon zest to taste

- 2–3 pinches salt

- ½ cup pitted dates, finely chopped

- 1 lb of whole blueberries of choice, can be combinations of berries

- Extra natural sweetener (optional)

Directions:

1. In a saucepan, add the dates, berries, and sea salt, then cook over medium-low heat.
2. Heat the mixture until it starts to bubble and the berries start to break apart.

3. Reduce the heat and let simmer with a cover for another 10 minutes to allow the fruit to completely break apart.

4. Add the lemon zest and chia and cook for another 3–5 minutes, allowing the chia to help thicken the jam.

5. Do a taste test and see if any sweetener is required.

6. Allow the jam to cool down completely before refrigerating.

Spinach-Walnut Pâté

Ingredients:

- ¼ cup fresh dill

- ¼ tsp coriander, ground

- ¼ cup fresh tarragon leaves

- 2 small cloves garlic, smashed

- 2 tbsp white wine vinegar

- 2 tbsp pomegranate seeds

- 1 ½ lbs fresh spinach, remove large stems

- ¾ cup walnuts, chopped and some extra for garnishing

- 3 scallions, chopped

- ½ cup fresh cilantro leaves

- Pinch cayenne pepper

- Salt to taste

- Crackers, for serving

Directions:

1. Add some plastic wrap to a 5-inch ramekin or small bowl, making sure that the plastic is as smooth as possible. Ensure that there is at least two inches extra overhang for the plastic.

2. Bring a pot of water to boil then add the spinach. It should be fully submerged. Cook for 1–2 minutes to allow the spinach to become tender and wilted.

3. Drain and dry the spinach thoroughly before chopping it finely. Place in a fresh bowl.

4. In a processor add ⅓ cup of warm water, dill, cilantro, tarragon, walnuts, coriander, vinegar, scallions, garlic, cayenne, and 1 ¼ teaspoon

salt, then blend until the mixture has the consistency of mayonnaise.

5. Stir this mixture in with the spinach and combine thoroughly. Spoon the mixture into the ramekin and pat down to compact it.

6. Cover with the overhanging plastic and refrigerate overnight.

7. Serve by unwrapping and upending the ramekin onto a fresh plate. Garnish with the pomegranate seeds and chopped walnuts left over.

8. Serve with pegan-friendly crackers, butternut toast, or vegetable sticks.

Potatoes For Breakfast

Ingredients:

- 3 medium potatoes, weighing approximately 400 grams (14 ounces);

- 2 tablespoons of olive oil

- 3 onions, medium size

- 2 teaspoon of ground cumin

- 8 ounces of extra-firm tofu (200g)

- 3 teaspoons of dried oregano

- 2 teaspoon of ground black pepper

- 2 teaspoon of table salt

- 1 a cup of cherry tomatoes (4 tomatoes)

Directions:

1. After washing the potatoes and chopping them into pieces around the size of your little finger, you should use the potatoes in this recipe.

2. The onions need to be peeled before being sliced into "half ring" pieces.

3. Heat a pan with a touch of olive oil, adjusting the heat to a setting between low and medium.

4. While the potatoes are cooking for the first five minutes, give them a light stirring every so often.

5. After the meat has begun to sweat, add the onions.

6. Crumble the tofu and add it at this point.

7. After that, salt and pepper are added while the mixture is being stirred. In that case, cover the pot and bring it to a simmer for fifteen minutes.

8. You could add more oil if it appears to be required, but if you want to cut down on the number of calories you take in, you could also add some hot water instead.

9. In a second pan, pour some olive oil into it, and then stir it around.

10. The temperature has been adjusted to medium.

11. After cutting the tomatoes in half lengthwise, they should be cooked for about five minutes, or until some black spots appear.

12. In addition to that, you can simmer a few drops of water that has been brought to a boil. Add salt and pepper to taste.

13. Place the potatoes on a tray, cover it, and place it in the oven if you do not have a second pan or if you do not wish to use it (or keep it warm in oven).

14. Arrange the tomato and potato mixture on a dish in a decorative manner.

Baked Oats

Ingredients:

- 3 cups of unsweetened coconut or almond milk in the measure of a cup

- 2-4 of a cup of pure maple syrup or unprocessed honey

- 1 tsp. extract from vanilla beans

- 2-4 cup of chopped nuts of your choice, such as almonds

- 1 tsp. of freshly grated lemon rind

- 1 banana (big), cut

- 4 eggs (large)

- 3 cups of oats that have been rolled

- 2-4 of a cup of protein powder in vanilla flavor

- Use coconut oil for lubricating the pan.

- 2 cup of mixed berries, either frozen or fresh.

Directions:

1. Preheat the oven to 350 degrees Fahrenheit and grease a 9x13 baking dish with coconut oil before placing it in the oven.

2. In a large mixing dish, eggs, honey, protein powder, vanilla extract, lemon zest, and milk should be mixed together until the mixture becomes foamy.

3. At this point, you should mix in your oats. To ensure that everything is thoroughly combined, stir it.

4. If you have the time, let the mixture sit for half an hour to allow the oats to absorb it.

5. After that, fold in the berries, banana slices, and almonds that have been roughly chopped.

6. After preparing the baking dish, pour the oat mixture into the prepared baking dish.

7. Bake for thirty to thirty-five minutes at a temperature of three hundred fifty degrees Fahrenheit, or until the center is firm and the top and edges are a golden brown color.

8. When the oats have achieved a beautiful golden brown color, remove them from the oven.

9. Cut the dough into six pieces or bars and evenly spread them apart.

10. Keeping these squares fresh for up to a week requires little more than placing them in a container with a tight-fitting lid and placing layers of wax paper in between them. They are good at heating up!

Green Smoothie

Ingredients:

- 1 organic mango

- 1 organic apple

- 1 organic banana

- juice of 1 organic lemon

- lemon peel

- 50 g chard

- 60 g spinach

- 2 ribs of celery

- 12 organic strawberries

- fresh spearmint

- 500 ml of water

Directions:

1. Wash and carefully clean the chard and spinach then tear the leaves into pieces.

2. Wash the celery and remove the filaments on the back with a small knife then cut into pieces.

3. Wash the strawberries, mint and apple, peel the mango and cut it into pieces.

4. Place all the INGREDIENTS: in the blender and operate.

5. Add the lemon zest last, blend and serve with fresh mint leaves!

Crepes With Red Fruits And Dried Fruits

Ingredients:

- 20 g coconut flour

- 70 g almond milk

- 200 g mixed red fruits (raspberries, wild strawberries, blueberries, blackberries, currants)

- Coconut oil

- 3 egg whites

- 60 g mixed nuts (hazelnuts, almonds, walnuts, pistachios)

- Stevia

Directions:

1. In a bowl, beat egg whites with coconut flour and milk until smooth then pour one ladle at a time onto a nonstick pan greased lightly with coconut oil and cook the crepes
2. Take the red berries, wash them and then cut them in half. In a pan pour 60 ml of water, stevia and the red fruits and let them soften for about 5 min. Stuff each crepe with the fruit "jam" and chopped nuts!

Chocolate Chip Cookies

Ingredients:

- 3 tbsp softened, cooled coconut oil

- ¼ cup and 2 tbsp maple syrup

- ¼ cup and 2 tbsp cassava flour

- ¼ cup and 2 tbsp almond flour

- 4 oz coarsely ambivalent (over 75% cocoa) chocolate, cleaved (have extra for the highest point of the cookies)

- ½ cup cashew margarine, at room

- temperature and well-stirred ½ tsp baking soda

- ¼ tsp salt, fine

- 1 tbsp coconut sugar

- 1 tsp vanilla extract

- flaky salt for sprinkling over the top

Directions:

1. Preheat the stove to 375 °F.

2. Set a rack to the upper third of the oven.

3. Line a treat sheet with material paper.

   In a bowl whisk the vanilla, cashew spread, coconut sugar, coconut oil,

4. and maple syrup until totally smooth.

   Sift the almond and cassava flours with the ocean salt and baking soft drink together.

5. Stir along with the chocolate chunks.

   Add the dry fixings to the wet and mix well.

6. Scoop sufficient mixture (around three tablespoons) to make one treat on the pre-arranged treat sheet.

   Keep the space between treats to 2-3 inches apart.

Place some chocolate on the highest point of the treat batter with a sprinkle of flaky salt.

7. Bake the treats on the top rack for 8-12 minutes or until they are brilliant and puffy

8. The edges ought to be set and the middle delicate and chewy.

9. To guarantee the treats heat equally, turn the baking plate at 8 minutes and go on for a couple of more minutes.

10. Once cooked, eliminate the treats, and put them on a wire rack and permit them to cool.

11. Cookies can be appreciated warm or cooled yet will just keep going for three days at room temperature.

12. Freeze once cooled on the off chance that you won't eat them immediately.

Chia Pudding With Almond Butter And Jam

Ingredients:

- 4 tbsp of any milk alternative

- 6 blueberries

- 4 raspberries

- 4 tsp of almond butter

- 8 tsp of custom made jam, pegan-friendly

- A couple of pistachios, chopped

- 1 tbsp of chia seeds

- 1 tbsp of flaxseed

Directions:

1. In a glass container that needs a cover, blend a tablespoon of flaxseed and chia to four tablespoons of milk.

2. Mix until every one of the seeds are totally drenched and allowed them to rest for two hours or shortterm in the fridge.

3. In a new glass container, add 2 teaspoons of jam, with 2 teaspoons of the chia and flaxseed pudding, 2 teaspoons of the almond margarine, then, at that point, one more 2 teaspoons of jam, trailed by what is left of the pudding.

4. Top with the berries and pistachios before serving.

Almond Berry Cobbler

Ingredients:

For berry filling:

- 1 tablespoon (20 g) maple syrup

- 1 teaspoon fresh lemon juice

- 1 vanilla bean, scraped (reserve the pod for another use, like in smoothies)

- 8 cups (1.2 kg) fresh mixed berries (I used 3 cups strawberries, 3 cups blueberries, and 2 cups blackberries)

- 2 tablespoons (16 g) arrowroot

For biscuit topping:

- ½ teaspoon almond extract

- ½ teaspoon sea salt ½ teaspoon baking soda

- 2 cups (192 g) blanched almond flour

- ¼ cup (32 g) arrowroot

- 1 large egg white, beaten (optional)

- ⅓ cup (31 g) raw sliced almonds

- ¼ cup (60 ml) unsweetened Almond Milk
  (here) or store-bought almond milk

- ¼ cup (56 g) coconut oil, melted

- 3 tablespoons (60 g) maple syrup

Directions:

1. Preheat the oven to 400°F (200°C, or gas mark
   6).

2. To make the berry filling: In a large bowl,
   combine the berries, arrowroot, maple syrup,
   lemon juice, and scraped vanilla bean seeds.
   Gently mix to coat the berries evenly. Transfer
   to an 8 × 8-inch (20 × 20 cm) baking dish.

3. To make the biscuit topping: In a medium-size bowl, whisk the almond milk, melted coconut oil, maple syrup, and almond extract to combine. Add the salt and baking soda and whisk again to incorporate.

4. Add the almond flour and arrowroot and use a spoon to mix the dry INGREDIENTS: into the wet INGREDIENTS:, until no dry INGREDIENTS: remain. Spoon the biscuit topping over the berries in 3 rows of 3 mounds. Use the spoon to gently mix up the topping and spread it over the top, making a rustic, uneven covering.

5. Brush the biscuits with the beaten egg white to make a beautiful shiny topping (if using).

6. Evenly sprinkle the almonds over the topping. Cover the baking dish with aluminum foil.

7. Bake the cobbler for 35 minutes, covered. Remove the foil and bake the cobbler for 12 to 15 minutes more until the topping is lightly

browned. Almond flour browns and burns quickly, so check on the cobbler before the end of the baking time.

8. Refrigerate leftovers tightly wrapped, or in an airtight container, for up to 4 days.

Vanilla-Poached Pears

Ingredients:

- 1 tablespoon (20 g) maple syrup

- 1 tablespoon (15 ml) fresh lemon juice

- 1 cinnamon stick

- 1 teaspoon grated lemon zest

- ¼ cup (28 g) chopped pecans

- 2 firm pears, any variety

- 1 vanilla bean

- 1½ cups (360 ml) water

- 1 cup (240 ml) sweet white wine, such as Moscato

Directions:

1. Halve the pears and cut out the core and seeds.

2. Leave the stem on the pears for presentation, if desired.

3. Halve the vanilla bean lengthwise so the seeds are exposed.

4. In a small skillet large enough to hold the pears in a single layer, over medium heat, arrange the pears halves and add the water, white wine, maple syrup, lemon juice, vanilla bean, cinnamon stick, and lemon zest. Bring to a simmer.

5. Cover the skillet and cook for 7 minutes. Remove the lid, flip the pears, and simmer for 7 minutes more to concentrate the syrup until it is reduced to about ½ cup (120 ml). If the syrup becomes too concentrated, thin it with a few tablespoons (about 45 ml) of water.

6. Serve the pears with a drizzle of the white wine syrup, topped with 1 tablespoon (7 g) of chopped pecans.

Cold Melon Balls With Mint

Ingredients:

- 1 tbsp. Honey

- 100 ml peach juice

- 1 melon cantaloupe or charentais

- 1 lime juice

- 1 orange juice

- Chopped mint for the garnish.

Directions:

1. Break the melon fifty-fifty, scratch the seeds, and cut 200 g little balls from the mash with a ball shaper and refrigerate them.

2. Remove the excess mash from the skin and cut it into enormous lumps prior to putting it in a cup.

3. Combine with the lime, orange and peach squeeze and mix all together.
4. If required, add some water to make a fine puree and refrigerate no less than 2 hour.
5. Split the puree on 4 dishes decorate with some melon balls and mint and serve.

Monkfish With Mediterranean Vegetables

Ingredients:

- 1 splash lemon juice 3

- Tbsps. Olive oil

- 1 yellow pepper

- 10 g chives (0.5 bunch)

- 500 g zucchini (2 zucchini) 720

- G monkfish fillet

- 1 green pepper

- 1 clove garlic

- 1 red pepper

- 1 shallot

- Pepper

- Sea-salt

Directions:

1. Wash, cored and cut peppers into cubes.

2. Peel and clove shallot and garlic and cleave them.

3. Put 2 tablespoons olive oil in a skillet and sauté shallot and garlic until clear over medium heat.

4. Cook for 2 minutes in the wake of adding the pepper solid shapes, then, at that point, deglazing with lemon juice. Season with salt and pepper.

5. Meanwhile, wash the chives and slice them into fine rolls.

6. Remove the pan from the heat and add the chives.

7. Cut the monkfish into 10 medallions, each about 1 inch thick and weighs 70 g.

8. Place medallions in a baking dish with vegetables. Season with salt and pepper.

9. Cook for about 10 minutes in a preheated oven at 160° C (fan oven: 140° C).

10. Meanwhile, wash, clean and cut the zucchini into thinly slices. 10. In a pan, heat 1 tablespoon of olive oil and sauté the zucchini for 2- 3 minutes, seasoning with salt.

11. Place 3 filled monkfish medallions on top of zucchini on 4 dish plates and serve.

Celery Mushroom Soup

Ingredients:

- 1 (8-ounce) package cremini mushrooms, sliced

- 1 medium bunch celery, trimmed and thinly sliced

- 6 cups Basic Vegetable Stock (see recipe in this chapter)

- 1 teaspoon dried thyme leaves

- 1 teaspoon salt

- 2 tablespoons olive oil

- 1 medium shallot, peeled and finely minced

- 1 / 8 teaspoon ground white pepper

- 1 tablespoon lemon juice

Directions:

1. In large pot, heat olive oil over medium heat.

2. Add shallot; cook until softened, about 3 minutes.

3. Add mushrooms; cook and stir until mushrooms give up their liquid, about 8 minutes.

4. Add celery and cook for 4 minutes longer. Add stock, thyme, salt, and white pepper, and bring to a simmer.

5. Cover pot, reduce heat to low, and simmer for 15–20 minutes or until soup is blended. Stir in lemon juice and serve immediately.

Carrot Lemon Soup

Ingredients:

- 6 cups Basic Vegetable Stock (see recipe in this chapter)

- 1 teaspoon minced fresh ginger

- Juice and zest from 1 large lemon

- 1 / 2 teaspoon ground black pepper

- 3 tablespoons olive oil

- 2 pounds carrots, peeled and diced

- 2 large yellow onions, peeled and diced

- 2 cloves garlic, peeled and minced

- 3 green onions, thinly sliced

Directions:

1. Heat olive oil in a large stockpot over medium heat.

2. Sauté carrots, yellow onions, and garlic until softened, about 8 minutes.

3. Add stock and bring to a boil over high heat.

4. Reduce heat to low and simmer for approximately 1 hour.

5. Add ginger, lemon juice, and zest. Season with pepper.

6. Garnish with green onions. Serve hot or refrigerate for at least 4 hours.

Sweet Red Salad With Chicken

Ingredients:

- 1 3 / 4 teaspoons salt, divided

- 3 / 4 teaspoon ground black pepper, divided

- 5 cups baby spinach

- 1 cup sliced strawberries

- 1 / 2 cup chopped pecans

- 2 tablespoons apple cider vinegar

- 2 tablespoons maple syrup

- 4 small beets, peeled and chopped

- 1 tablespoon plus 1 / 4 cup olive oil, divided

- 1 pound boneless, skinless chicken breast

- 2 tablespoons orange juice

Directions:

1. Place beets in a medium saucepan and cover with water.

2. Boil beets in water until soft, about 20 minutes. Drain beets and allow to cool completely.

3. Meanwhile, heat 1 tablespoon olive oil in a large nonstick frying pan over medium heat. Season both sides of chicken with 3 / 4 teaspoon salt and 1 / 4 teaspoon pepper.

4. Add chicken to the pan. Cover the pan and cook until just cooked through, 5–8 minutes on each side.

5. Transfer chicken to a cutting board and let cool.

6. Cut the chicken into bite-sized pieces.

7. In a large bowl, combine chicken, spinach, strawberries, pecans, and cooled beets.

8. In a separate small bowl, whisk together remaining olive oil, vinegar, maple syrup, and

orange juice, and pour over salad, tossing well to coat.

9. Season with remaining salt and black pepper.

Tangerine, Mint, And Quinoa Salad

Ingredients:

- 2 tablespoons chopped fresh mint

- 2 large tangerines, peeled and sectioned

- 1 / 3 cup chopped walnuts

- 1 bulb fennel, thinly sliced

- 2 tablespoons olive oil

- 1 teaspoon salt

- 1 cup uncooked quinoa

- 2 cups water

- 1 medium head green leaf lettuce, chopped

- 1 / 2 teaspoon ground black pepper

Directions:

1. Fill medium pot with water, add quinoa and bring to a boil.

2. When water boils, reduce heat to low and cover; simmer 15 minutes.

3. Remove from heat and keep covered an additional 5 minutes; then fluff with a fork and set aside.

4. Gently toss together quinoa, lettuce, mint, tangerines, walnuts, and sliced fennel.

5. Drizzle with olive oil, season with salt and black pepper, and serve immediately.

Ribbon Salad

Ingredients:

- 2 medium yellow summer squash

- 2 tablespoons olive oil

- 3 tablespoons lemon juice

- 1 tablespoon Dijon mustard

- 1 tablespoon chopped fresh dill

- 1 / 2 teaspoon salt

- 2 medium zucchini

- 2 large carrots, peeled

- 1 / 8 teaspoon ground black pepper

Directions:

1. Rinse vegetables and pat dry; cut off ends.

2. Using a vegetable peeler or a mandoline, shave vegetables into thin, wide ribbons.

3. Don't use the seedy cores of the zucchini and squash; discard those when you get to them.

4. In a large bowl, combine olive oil, lemon juice, mustard, dill, salt, and black pepper and mix well.

5. Add vegetable ribbons and toss to coat.

6. Serve immediately, or cover and refrigerate for up to 24 hours before serving.

Marinated Flank Steak

Ingredients:

Marinade:

- 2 tablespoons fresh lemon juice

- 1 ½ tablespoon Worcestershire sauce

- 1tablespoon Dijon mustard

- 2cloves garlic, minced

- ½ teaspoon ground black pepper

- ½ cup vegetable oil

- ⅓ cup low-sodium soy sauce

- ¼ cup red wine vinegar

Steak:

- 1 (1 1/2-pound) flank steak

Directions:

1. In a 9x13-inch glass baking dish, add oil, soy sauce, vinegar, lemon juice, Worcestershire sauce, Dijon mustard, garlic, and pepper for marinating.

2. In a baking dish, add flank steak and toss several times to coat it in the marinade.

3. Taking the lid off and put it in the fridge for 2 to 6 hours, or longer if you have the time.

4. A medium-high outdoor grill should be preheated and lightly oiled before cooking.

5. The excess marinade should be shaken off the steak before it is taken out of the marinade.

6. Throw away any leftover marinade.

7. To get the appropriate doneness, cook steak on a hot grill for about 5 minutes on each side.

8. Before cutting and serving the meat, let it to rest for 5 minutes.

Grilled Marinated Flank Steak

Ingredients:

Marinade INGREDIENTS:

- 2 cloves garlic, minced

- 2 tablespoons red wine vinegar

- 1/3 cup soy sauce

- 1/4 cup honey

- 1/3 cup extra virgin olive oil

- 1/2 teaspoon freshly ground black pepper

Other INGREDIENTS:

- 1(2-pound) flank steak

- Coarse salt, to taste (optional)

- More freshly ground black pepper, to taste

117

Directions:

1. Prepare the marinade in a large non-reactive basin.Turn the steak in the marinade to coat it fully. (Alternatively, throw the steak and marinate in a freezer bag and freeze.)

2. Marinate for 2 hours or overnight.

3. marinade in a glass

4. Prepare your grill for high direct heat and low indirect heat. The grill is hot enough when you hold your palm an inch over the scorching side for a second.

5. Griddle the steak: Remove it from the marinade and carefully shake off the excess marinade (but leave enough marinade to keep it from adhering to the grill).

6. If desired, season with coarse salt and freshly ground pepper. A delicious crust on the steak from the salt and pepper.

7. Place steak on the hot grill side. Grill for a fewer minutes on each side to sear. Continue

cooking the steak for a few minutes longer until it is done to your preference.

8. Remove the steak from the grill and set it on a cutting board to rest. Cover with aluminum foil to keep the steak warm for 10–15 minutes.

9. Slice against the grain: The orientation of the steak's muscle fibers is termed the meat's grain. Flank steak is a lean cut that may be rough and chewy if not sliced properly.

10. So, cut the steak on a steep diagonal so the pieces are broad. I like a long serrated bread knife, but any long sharp knife would suffice.

Baked Halibut Delight

Ingredients:

- 1 onion, chopped

- 5 ounces kalamata olives, pitted

- ¼ cup capers

- ¼ cup olive oil

- 1 tablespoon lemon juice

- 6 ounces halibut fillets

- 1 tablespoon Greek seasoning

- 1 large tomato, chopped

- Salt and pepper as needed

Directions:

1. Preheat your oven to 350 degrees Fahrenheit

2. Transfer the halibut fillets on a large aluminum foil

3. Season with Greek seasoning

4. Take a bowl and add tomato, onion, olives, olive oil, capers, pepper, lemon juice, and salt

5. Mix well and spoon the tomato mix over the halibut

6. Seal the edges and fold to make a packet

7. Place the packet on a baking sheet and bake in your oven for 30-40 minutes

8. Serve once the fish flakes off, and enjoy!

9. Serve over rice cauliflower if desired

Avocado Stuffed With Pico De Gallo

Ingredients:

- 1 tbsp lime juice, freshly squeezed

- 1 ½–2 tbsp cilantro, minced

- ½ tsp salt

- 1 tbsp jalapeño, minced (optional)

- 3 medium/large avocado

- 2 Roma tomatoes, diced

- 3 tbsp onions, diced

Directions:

1. Prepare the tomatoes, onions, cilantro, and jalapeño (optional).

2. In a large bowl, mix the prepared vegetables and sprinkle with salt and lime juice before stirring well—this is the pico de gallo.

3. Cut the avocados in half and remove the seeds.
4. Widen and deepen the seed holes scooping at the sides with a spoon. The larger the hole the more it can be stuffed.
5. Fill the scooped-out holes with the pico de gallo.
6. Serve fresh to prevent the avocado from turning brown.

Stuffed Peppers

Ingredients:

- 1 handful fresh basil

- 18 oz cherry tomatoes

- 3 tbsp olive oil

- 3 fresh garlic cloves

- 2 tbsp balsamic vinegar

- 4 red bell pepper

- 2 shallots

- Salt to taste

- Freshly ground pepper to taste

Directions:

1. Cut the bell peppers in half lengthwise then remove the ribs and the seeds.

2. Brush the outside of the pepper with some oil and season with salt.

3. Then, arrange the peppers cut-side down on a baking pan and grill in the oven for 8–10 minutes.

4. Clean the shallots and tomatoes.

5. Cut the tomatoes in half, peel the garlic and shallots, then cut both finely.

6. Chop the basil leaves finely. Add all the INGREDIENTS: to a bowl.

7. Drizzle the contents of the bowl with 2 tablespoons of oil and balsamic vinegar then mix well.

8. Do a taste test before seasoning with salt and pepper.

9. Remove the peppers from the oven and brush the sides with the remaining oil before filling the center with the stuffing.

10. Return the peppers to the oven and grill for another five minutes.

11. Serve immediately with some fresh basil as garnish.

Salad With Tacos And Grilled Chicken

Ingredients:

- 2 tablespoons of chili powder;

- 1 tablespoon of lime juice;

- 1 teaspoon of powdered cumin;

- 1 teaspoon of ground coriander;

- 14 teaspoon of cayenne pepper;

- 2 pound of chicken breast halves that have been boned and skinned

- 2 tablespoon of olive oil

- 5 corn tortillas measuring seven inches in diameter

- One-half cup of finely chopped fresh cilantro • Four cups of shredded lettuce

- 2 avocado that has been peeled, pitted, and sliced (Optional)

- a quarter cup of salsa with a medium level of heat

- 1 can of black beans (15 ounces), washed and drained;

- 1/2 cup of chopped fresh cilantro;

- Optional: a quarter cup of sour cream

- Required: one lime, sliced into wedges (Optional)

Directions:

1. Preheat an outside grill to medium-high heat and lightly oil the grate surfaces before beginning to cook.

2. Mix the black beans, salsa, lime juice, and half of the cilantro together in a bowl and set aside.

3. To season chicken breasts with this mixture, combine chili powder, coriander, cumin, brown sugar, olive oil, and cayenne pepper in a bowl.

4. Then, rub the mixture onto the chicken breasts.

5. Place the chicken breasts on a grill over medium-high heat for ten to twelve minutes per side, or until the juices run clear and the center is no longer pink.

6. A thermometer with an instant readout should register at least 165 degrees Fahrenheit in the centre (74 degrees C).

7. Put the tortillas on the grill and cook them for three to five minutes, or until they are just beginning to get a little bit of a golden color on both sides.

8. After transferring the chicken to a chopping board, cut it into thin, long strips using a sharp knife.

9. Place the chicken strips, the bean mixture, the lettuce, and the remaining half cup of cilantro on top of the tortillas and mix everything together.

10. Avocado, sour cream, and lime wedges should be served alongside this dish.

Kale Smoothie

Ingredients:

- 1 tablespoon peanut butter

- 1 tablespoon chia seeds

- 1 banana

- 2 oz. spinach leaves

- 1 cup soy milk

Directions:

1. In a blender place all INGREDIENTS: and blend until smooth

2. Pour smoothie in a glass and serve

Green Juice Smoothie

Ingredients:

- 1 cucumber

- ½ cup kale leaves

- ¼ lemon

- 2 apples

- 2 celery sticks

Directions:

1. In a blender place all INGREDIENTS: and blend until smooth
2. Pour smoothie in a glass and serve

Chicken Schnitzel With Zucchini Strips

Ingredients:

- 4 tbsps. Olive oil

- ½ lemon (juice)

- Pepper

- 2 garlic cloves

- 1000 g zucchini (4 zucchini)

- 10 g basil (0.5 bunch)

- 700 g chicken breast fillet (4 chicken breast fillets) 2 branches rosemary

- 4 branches thyme

- Sea-salt

- 160 g tomatoes (2 tomatoes)

Directions:

1. Rinse the chicken fillets under cold water, and pat dry. After that, knock out thinly.

2. Wash, peel and chop f finely the garlic, basil, rosemary, and thyme.

3. Combine 2 tablespoons of olive oil, half of the garlic, lemon juice, rosemary, thyme, and pepper in a small mixing bowl.

4. In a large baking dish layer the meat and pour the marinade over it and let rest for at least 3 hours.

5. Meanwhile, Clean and wash the zucchini before cutting it lengthwise into slices of 3 mm wide approx.

6. Mix in the remaining 2 tbsp of oil with garlic, salt, and pepper, and pour the marinade over zucchini and let rest.

7. Scald tomatoes in boiling water for 3 minutes, put them into cold water then peel and cut

into small cubes. Season with a pinch of salt and pepper.

8. Remove the chicken from the marinade, season with salt, and grill for 2 minutes on both sides on a hot grill or in a preheated grill pan.

9. Place the zucchini in a pan with the marinade and cook for 2 minutes over medium heat, or until al dente.

10. Place the chicken breast fillets on four preheated plates whit zucchini and garnish with diced tomatoes.

Cashew Hot Fudge

Ingredients:

- 2 tablespoons (28 g) coconut oil

- 2 tablespoons (40 g) maple syrup or date syrup

- Pinch sea salt

- 6 tablespoons (98 g) cashew butter

- 6 tablespoons (30 g) cacao powder (see note)

- 3 tablespoons (45 ml) avocado oil

Directions:

1. In a small saucepan, whisk all the INGREDIENTS: to combine well. If your coconut oil is solid, don't worry. It will melt into the sauce in the next step.

2. Place the saucepan over low heat, and cook, whisking, for about 5 minutes until the sauce is melted, warmed, and easily whisks together. It does not need to bubble.

3. Store leftovers at room temperature. The sauce will thicken when it cools, so reheat it before using again.

4. I like to store it in a glass jar and put the glass jar in hot water for 5 to 10 minutes, stirring it well halfway through the heating time. If necessary, thin it with more coconut oil.

Sneaky Black Bean Brownies

Ingredients:

- 2 teaspoons pure vanilla extract

- 1/3 cup ground flaxseed

- 1 large pasture-raised egg

- 1/3 cup pure maple syrup

- 1 tablespoon granulated monk fruit sweetener, for baking (optional)

- ¼ teaspoon sea salt

- 1 (15-ounce) can low-sodium black beans

- ¼ avocado

- 1 tablespoon coconut oil, melted

- 2 tablespoons nut butter (preferably cashew butter)

- ½ teaspoon baking powder

- 1/3 cup unsweetened organic cacao powder

- ½ cup dairy-free dark chocolate chips (preferably sweetened with monk fruit or stevia)

Directions:

1. Drain the beans and rinse them well, letting them dry in a sieve.
2. Preheat the oven to 350°F. Line an 8 x 8-inch baking dish with parchment paper.
3. Place the avocado, coconut oil, nut butter, vanilla extract, and beans in a food processor.
4. Blend for 30 seconds until combined. Scrape the sides if needed.

5. Add the ground flaxseed, egg, maple syrup, monk fruit (if using), salt, and baking powder and process for 20 seconds.

6. Sift the cacao powder into the food processor bowl and process for 10 seconds. Scrape the sides and process for another 5 seconds. The batter should be thick and sticky.

7. Spread half of the mixture in the baking dish, sprinkle on the chocolate chips, and spread the rest of the batter on top. Smooth evenly with a spatula or the back of a spoon.

8. Place the baking dish on the top rack of the oven and bake for 25 minutes, or until the center of the brownie in the pan no longer jiggles. If testing with a toothpick, the toothpick should come out a bit sticky for fudgy brownies.

9. Remove from the oven and let cool completely before slicing into 14 pieces. Store

leftovers in an airtight container in the fridge for up to 5 days.